What People *In The Know* Are Saying About

52 Vitality TOOLS

"The world's health consciousness is shifting from a focus on treating disease to a focus on enhancing vitality. At birth, we were never given an instruction manual to help us optimize our life experience. Dr. Bruck has written just such a manual here. I highly recommend that you read, apply, and share!"

Liam P. Schubel DC
Schubel Vision Worldwide
www.schubelvisionworldwide.com

"I love this book! The concepts in it are in bite sized pieces and you can easily take on one at a time. These steps really are vital! We have unknowingly and unwittingly become a nation of powerless sick people and here in this book you are given a blueprint for living a more ALIVE life. Follow the easy-to-apply guidelines, and then you finally look in the mirror and say, `I AM doing good things for myself!' There is no greater feeling and it is what you were designed for! You were not designed to walk around half alive. A vital book!"

Dr. Pam Jarboe
Speaker, writer and c

What People *In The Know* Are Saying About

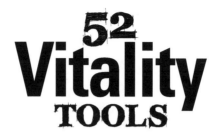

"Dr. Jenny makes it easier for you to get healthy. Her work is always informative, effective and inspiring. In this Internet Age, she knows that people don't need more information—they need transformation. Once again, she delivers in typical fashion. Easy to read, easy to follow, Jenny is always there—leading from the front—ready with a hug, a high-five or a head-lock—whatever will help you succeed."

Dr. Stephen Franson
Founder and CEO of Bonfire Health, Inc.
and MVP360 Coaching

"After twenty five years of teaching natural healing principles and personal development training around the world, this is a book I would have wanted to write. These 52 'tools' aren't just good ideas, rather the stepping stones to leading an extraordinary life."

Dr. CJ Mertz
CEO and President of CJ3 Consulting, LLC

"Thank you Dr. Jenny for inspiring each of us to listen to our innate intelligence. Everyone needs to hear the truth that their body functions best and expresses more life potential when there are no detrimental interferences to the nervous system."

Dr. Edwin Cordero
President of Sherman College of Chiropractic

"A Colleague, close friend and holistic health partner, Dr.Jenny and I have worked closely to help our clients and community learn the simplicity of staying healthy. Her book *52 Vitality Tools* gives the reader all the necessary practical gems to "heal" from the inside out! Read one tool per week, or drink in all the knowledge at once and spend the next 52 weeks, 52 months and 52 years engaging in vitality! This book is brilliant and can and will guide you back into balance! My favorite is number one and number 41, "Stop the Fear" and "Do What You Love!"

Dr. Margrit Mikulis
Naturopathic Doctor, Ayurvedic Practitioner and Executive Board Secretary of the National Ayurvedic Medical Association.

Jenny Bruck's *52 Vitality Tools* is a must read for anyone that is trying to improve their health. It is set up so you can apply one tip per week to create the new you in just 52 weeks. Simply put — an easy to read owner's manual for the human body.

Dr. Billy Demoss
Founder of Dead Chiropractic Society and California Jam

"A fantastically practical owner's manual to your body. Everyone should read this. Straight forward, thought provoking and full of wisdom. *52 Vitality Tools* is perfect for learning how to work with your body naturally to promote health, healing and radiant vitality."

Dr. Stephanie Mills
Ms. America 2014

This publication contains the opinions and ideas of the author. It is intended to provide helpful and informative material on the subjects addressed in the publication. It is sold with the understanding that the author and publisher are not engaged in rendering medical, health, psychological, or any other kind of personal professional services in the book. If the reader requires personal health assistance or advice, a competent professional should be consulted.

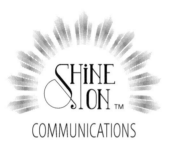

Published by

Shine On Communications
1 Overlook Dr. #7
03031

Copyright © 2014, 2015 by Dr. Jenny Bruck
Cover photograph by AlyssaKate Photography

Manufactured in the United States of America

For discounts on bulk purchases please contact us through our website at ShineOnCommunications.com

ISBN-13: 978-1496000385
ISBN-10: 1496000382

52 Vitality TOOLS

Daily Habits To Build Your *Bounce*

Dr. Jenny Bruck

*For two of the most essential
and energetic people in my life:
Mom and Dad.*

52
Vitality
TOOLS

Contents

Contents

Forward

by David E. Altobelli, D.M.D., M.D.

Biomedical Engineer
Oral and Maxillofacial Surgeon
Certified Personal Trainer
Certified Health Coach and Owner - UltraVitality, LLC

When I think of vitality, I think of physical and mental strength and vigor with boundless energy to be, do and have what I aspire. It's the energy to climb that mountain, to tackle that challenging project, to keep up with your kids, or to have enough energy at the end of the day to volunteer for that needy cause.

With vitality, you have motivation to do things--a lot of things--rather than constantly think about resting, eating or sleeping. And it's about more than just being "healthy," which often in our current health care system means "not being sick." We all have had our vital signs taken (blood pressure, pulse, respiratory rate, and temperature). Yes, when you have been injured or are very sick, they are important metrics of your health. However, they all can be within "normal limits," yet you don't have the energy to get off the couch!

When your vitality is low, the road of life feels as if it's a constant uphill climb. Everything seems to take effort. It's difficult to make decisions. Your motivation is low and you narrow your ambitions because you can't trust yourself to complete even simple tasks. You minimize the extent and scope of your activities. Often, all you can think about is just trying to get yourself through the day. Rather than thriving, you desperately try to survive.

Wouldn't it be magnificent if the road of life always felt

like pedaling a bicycle downhill? You would have the energy to experience the extraordinary joy in living *(joie de vivre)* and, with every day, you would be ready to seize the moment *(carpe diem)*. You'd have passion in what you do, and you could trust yourself to get things done. The day would seem as if it were giving you more time to accomplish all your goals. You could live your life with gusto and get all the "juice" out of what being human and alive has to offer. You truly could be happy and fulfilled, and it would be contagious to those around you. The world simply looks like a better and brighter place when your mind and body are in a state of high vitality. Wow...is this really possible?

Wherever you fall in the spectrum of vitality, Dr. Bruck's book of fifty-two vitality tools gives you the elements you need to either move your current vitality to a higher level, or to metaphorically reboot your system. With years of experience caring for patients, giving workshops, sharing her knowledge through radio shows, and presenting at national meetings, Dr. Bruck has the experience, depth of knowledge, and compassion to motivate patients to take action and make real and positive changes.

This book covers the fundamental — and essential — concepts in nutrition, sleep, exercise, ergonomics, a healing mindset, and how to live with intent/purpose.

These building blocks of vitality are presented as clear and concise concepts or tools that allow you to quickly take action to develop your own stable and vibrant infrastructure of health. These vitality elements can be implemented in the order they are presented. Or you may find that some of the tools may concentrate on your most current needs and you can focus on those that apply to your unique situation. Dr. Bruck wants these modules to resonate with your own personal growth and help you to identify with where you need to start taking action now!

We're all accustomed to our current medical model and believe the solution to our health problems must come from the outside, such as surgery and pharmaceuticals. I think most patients are now catching on and realizing that the real solutions for change come from within.

Our bodies have intrinsic intelligence: it starts with two cells and creates an exquisite human body with over forty trillion cells. The key is to give our bodies the nutrients that it needs and to take away what is toxic and blocking normal function. It is well known that our lifestyle — eating, exercise, stress, sleep, and social habits — is responsible for over eighty percent of the chronic diseases of our time from cardiovascular disease, cancer, respiratory diseases, to diabetes. Our food has the greatest influence on our health and the ability of our body to function as it was intended. The more whole, natural, and nutrient rich the food is in our diet, the more normally our bodies can function. Food is more than just calories; it is nutrition and information that speaks to our genes to express our biochemistry and function. These important dietary keys to health are concisely covered in this book's toolbox.

A journey of a thousand miles begins with a single step, according to the Chinese phlosopher Lao-Tzu (604-531 BC). By taking on each small, simple, but strategic step outlined by Dr. Bruck, you will find yourself quickly moving toward your destination of vitality. How would your life be different if you had abundant physical and mental energy? How would you change your life and the lives of your family and friends? How would you change the world?

As Dr. Bruck informs us, it's in the process that you will find happiness and fulfillment. Enjoy the journey!

52
Vitality
TOOLS

Introduction

People with smile lines have always attracted me. Even when they're serious, you can tell they smile often by the creases fanning their eyes and mouth. A spring in their step and a light in their soul usually accompany this vibrant expression. If you add a healthy physique, glowing skin and bright eyes, this is my snapshot vision of vitality.

I recently met an eighty-year-old woman who matched this description. Just being around her made me feel happy. I wanted to interview her, to get to know her. People who exude vitality have a magnetic quality about them. Their exuberance, confidence, and warmth make them special and rare. You'll find these dynamic individuals of any age, race, occupation or affluence. In general, they take extra care of their bodies and mind with a deliberate intention of improving themselves and maximizing their life experience. I often see families experiencing a state of vitality together as a lifestyle choice. They focus on physical activity, personal growth and purposeful choices for health. Instead of life happening to them, they create their level of fulfillment, energy and gusto.

Contrast this with the average person: overweight, on medication for preventable conditions, eating fast food, disliking their job, and tired all the time.

The curious thing is that we are not born with a manual on how to live healthy. We learn from our family, teachers and the media. Eventually, we may do our own studying through magazines, books and online research. Few people can say they were raised with parents who were natural health gurus. Even with the best of intentions, our generation's parents just didn't have abundant access to much of the information available today. On the flip side, many healthy choices are inherently obvious, yet an over-abundance of conflicting information has eroded our common sense. We struggle to trust our instincts. The task of listening to our body, sorting through inconsistent health information, knowing what to believe and deciphering what's most important is a gigantic undertaking. It's no wonder that optimal health and vitality eludes most folks. It's just too hard to figure out.

In practice, I've heard certain questions repeatedly. What links the questions together, whether they involve health philosophy, nutrition, sleep, exercise or ergonomics, is the intent. People just want to have more vitality. They want to feel well, look healthy, and function at their best. When asking about health goals, practice members will most often comment that they want to eat better and exercise more so they can feel and look younger and more alive. This has been my consistent observation over seventeen years in practice, and I'm not surprised. That's the outcome I strive for in my choices: vitality.

My idea for this book started when a practice member mentioned that she wished she had time to attend all my workshops or listen to all my radio shows. "Can't you just download the most important points to my brain?" she joked. The idea presented itself, and I was off.

Writing short quips about ways to increase vitality instead of a lengthy manual was born from the knowledge that most people aren't interested in purchasing and reading an entire book on a certain topic. For example, I often get questions such as "What is the best sleeping position?" or "How can I change my metabolism so I lose weight more easily?" People want quick answers; in effect a summation of all advice and research; something they can apply immediately. When it comes to living with more ease and vigor, people don't want to take a weekend course. They just want to know.

Introduction

In the following pages, I present the most vital information from the hundreds of workshops, radio shows and seminars I have given. I have downloaded the meatiest and most memorable information into 52 tools that, if employed, would certainly start you on a giant transformation toward vitality. You can read this book from cover to cover or just open up to a random page. Here's another option: I intentionally created 52 tools so you can contemplate one rule a week, implementing those that make your inner voice say "yes!" I promise this process will rebuild your bounce.

You'll find advice on nutrition, sleep, exercise, ergonomics, healing mindset and how to live intentionally. Some of this may appear common sense and obvious (yet an encouraging reminder) and others may surprise you. You may find a tool points to a path of study you would like to investigate. Tools that resonate with your own personal growth will attract you. Interestingly, if you pick up this book again a few months later, a different tool may leap out at you.

A giant chasm of support, resources and dedication separates knowing what to do and actually doing it. When I give a workshop on healthy living habits, the worst thing a participant can tell me is how interesting my talk was. Or that I did a good job. This level of influence does not change lives. What I want the participant to say is, "I know exactly what I need to do differently and I'm starting now."

Enjoy the process of growth and inspiration. Remember, each tool at one point was likely an entire seminar, so each paragraph is steeped in possibility. Feel free to ponder the significance a seemingly small change can make in the course of your life. True vitality springs from the compilation of an abundance of fine choices over the course of time.

I recognize that vitality is unbelievably multi-layered and

dynamic. I, for one, rarely keep all the balls in the air at once, and often find myself "re-starting" a commitment to my health. This, in actuality, is how vitality works. You don't achieve vitality, you re-create it every day.

Chances are, there has been a time in your life when you felt exceptionally vital. Vitality can be lost and then found often in a lifetime. I've always appreciated the concept that the journey is what creates happiness (see tool number forty three). The value is in creating vitality. True personal gratitude can happen from the life's work of taking care of yourself. Love yourself as you would your own child. Each fresh choice to apply a "tool" is a decision to love yourself. This is where vitality weaves its thread of spark into your life.

There's a reason I changed the original title of 52 Vitality Rules to 52 Vitality Tools.

Rules don't work if you're a person who tends to buck authority. I encourage this book to be thought of as a compilation of suggestions, guidelines, tips ... tools. Imagine you're speaking with a trusted old friend who gives you a little piece of advice. Sometimes an innocuous idea is just what you need to hear. The idea precipitates a change of thought, a reconsideration of habit, and ultimately a transformation. That is what I've experienced with practice members over the years at the adjusting table.

If you are not happy with your current level of health or vitality, perhaps you just have had the wrongs tools. If you have relied on "outside-in" solutions (medication, creams, potions and lotions for example) to look and feel well instead of consistent life habits that promote health, your toolbox is lacking. Let's explore some "inside-out" ideas to liven up your life. Ready, set, go!

About the Illustrations

The illustrations in this book are silhouettes representing physical tools you might use in different areas of your life — from the arts to industry and from the garden to personal care.

The silhouettes are placed throughout the book randomly. No connection is intended between the illustration on the left and the less tangible strategic or tactical tool I present on the right.

Dr. Jenny Bruck

Stop The Fear

We are raised to live in fear of germs. Now, I'm not saying there isn't an obvious value in washing your hands or refraining from making out with your sick, feverish partner, but fearing germs is futile. If you try to give someone a "cold," you'll need more than a virus to accomplish the job. Experimenters have incubated cold viruses, placed them directly on the mucus lining of the nose, and found that their subjects came down with colds only 12% of the time (1). Your body actually harbors most of the organisms you fear. It's like the trash: when it's all firmly bundled up on the curb, there's no problem. If the bag falls over, rips, and the trash falls out—then the bugs show up. The bugs were always around, but rallied and wreaked havoc once the trash appeared. The same goes with your body: we collect all sorts of harmless bacteria that don't cause illness unless we've created a junky environment. The question is this: Am I working toward cleaning up my body or am I creating a dump?

1. Chopra D. Quantum Healing. New York: Bantam Books. 1989;142.

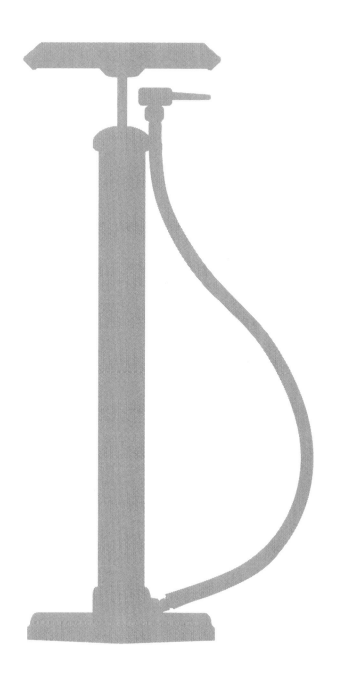

Know Symptoms Are Not Disease

"I have a cough." "I have a rash." "My child has a fever." We often (without even meaning to) label a symptom as the actual problem. A cough, a rash, or a fever is not the problem. In fact, it is the cure for the problem. When your body is working to adapt and heal, it creates ways to push out or burn off the bug or virus. The cough, rash and fever are all part of your body's amazing healing ability. Instead of having a knee-jerk reaction of overpowering this healing with a man-made, outside-in interference (i.e. drug), first evaluate if you can support the healing your body is already doing. The question is this: How can I support my healing right now, without interfering?

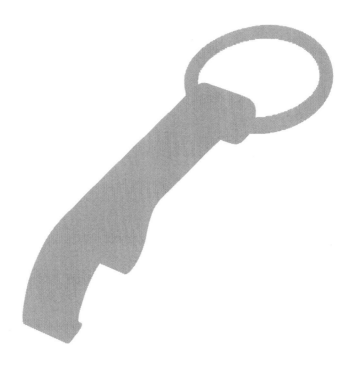

Slow Down to Heal

Being sick doesn't feel good. It's supposed to be that way. You are supposed to slow down, climb into bed and sleep. Healing occurs when you rest. If you ignore this simple fact and go about your busy life anyway, you'll prolong the healing time. Feel like you can't take the luxury of time to honor your healing needs? That's a sign that something might need to change in your life. Deciding that your health holds a high value for you means developing strategies to allow time for creating health... and time to heal when your body is sick. The question is this: Do I value my health enough to allow rest for healing?

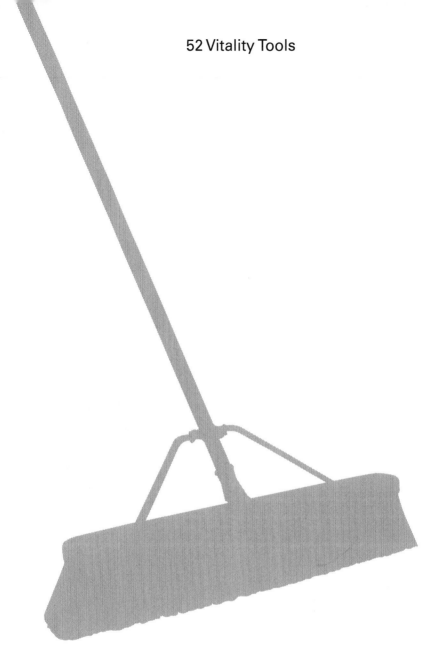

Clean Up Your "Healing" Language

When we are "sick," we naturally want to complain and list all our symptoms. A better way to refer to this healing process is as a "project." For example: "My body has a healing project right now. It's created a rash to push out what it doesn't want. Right now I'm using natural ways to support my healing while I figure out what caused the need for a rash." Your body always attempts to heal. Instead of seeing your body as failing you, honor your magnificent inner healing intelligence, starting with your words. Words have power. Especially with children. I know many children who are savvy in this language, and they speak powerfully about their body's healing ability. For example, one seven-year-old girl recently said to me, "I have a fever that is helping me heal. My body is strong." The question is this: Can I trust in my own healing ability, and speak words of this affirmation?

Find The Cause

No one ever got sick because they had a deficiency in a pharmaceutical drug. Even if you need "crisis" care, your next thought should be, "What caused this?" I'm not saying the answer will be obvious, or even possible to determine, but if you can figure it out (and there will likely be more than one cause), then you have the framework to create a healthier body. The only two causes of any illness are toxicity or deficiency. Examples of toxicity are chemicals in food, environment, or drugs (pushed or prescribed). Examples of deficiency are lack of movement (exercise), dehydration, lack of nutrients, or subluxation. The question is this: What toxicity or deficiency caused these symptoms of healing?

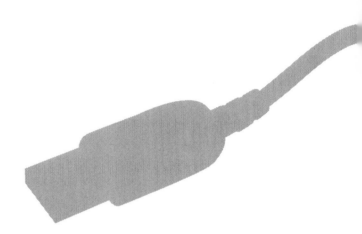

Do The Inside-Out Work

There is a saying in chiropractic that goes, "All healing happens from above-down-inside-out." Most people have been conditioned to the false concept of outside-in healing. Just look at all the drug advertisements on television. They say to take something from outside of you to fix you. Even natural products still have this overall mindset. I'm not suggesting that you should or shouldn't take that vitamin C capsule when you have a cold, but assess your habits as well. For example, do you think you can forgo exercise and just lie around and take protein powder to build muscles? Of course not. Yet radio and television shopping networks are flooded with the next quick fix. The work is simple: eat less, move more, think right, sleep well and keep your body aligned. No pill, potion, lotion or gadget can make up for the lack of these required "life nutrients." The question is this: Are my habits allowing me to heal from the inside-out?

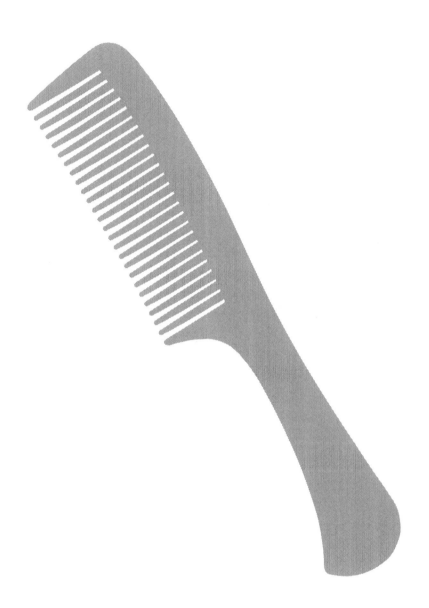

Repair Your Body

I'm sure you would agree that the benefit of eating healthfully happens when you actually do it. Once you stop, you rapidly lose the benefit. The same holds true for exercising, oral hygiene, taking nutritional supplements, wellness chiropractic adjustments and smart sleeping strategies. Once you're on track and reaping the rewards of "right" living, you are smartest to continue. You understand that you get out of it what you put into it. It all seems so simple, yet can be difficult to live by. Think of it this way: our bodies are always breaking down. Due to environmental forces, we can't escape this fact. How swiftly and aggressively we choose to repair this breakdown determines our health. If we are breaking down faster than we are repairing, then we create dis-ease. If we are repairing faster than we are breaking down, we create wellness. Vitality happens when we are repairing much faster than we are breaking down. The question is this: Are my lifestyle choices supporting my body's breakdown or its repair?

8

Re-connect and Replenish Nerve Flow

Did you know your spine is the house for your spinal cord? Just like your skull protects your priceless brain, your spine protects the spinal cord and nerve roots. Information flows from your brain out through the nerves to your whole body. This nerve power controls all function: immune system, heart, lungs, kidneys, stomach, intestines, etc. When the spine is unhealthy, these communication pathways can distort. A healthy spine allows the nerve system to do its job. Chiropractic may be known for helping neck and back pain, but families who utilize regular spinal check-ups for overall health experience benefits beyond expectations. My clinical observation over the years shows families who get adjusted regularly are sick less often, get well faster, have less symptoms (headaches, asthma, allergies, intestinal problems, infertility, earaches, etc.) and more energy and vitality. Here's the big picture: chiropractic is not a treatment for a condition or symptom. Rather, by removing nerve stress, adjustments allow your body to better work as designed. Celebrities, professional athletes and probably your neighbor know this. The question is this: Who's my chiropractor?

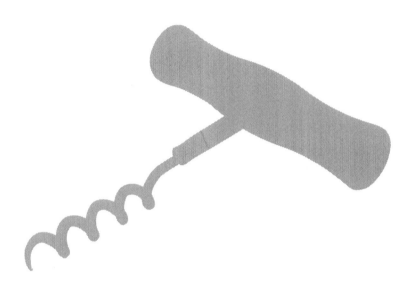

Sleep To Heal

During sleep, your body releases the hormone cortisol, which helps to boost your immune system. Notice how you feel more tired when you're sick? This is because your immune system releases chemicals called cytokines when you have an infection. These chemicals induce sleep so your body can heal. When ill, fever tends to happen when sleeping; again, this is your body's healing mechanisms shifting into high gear for you. A good night's sleep and even a nap during the day will help your body overcome illness. Even when you don't have an obvious healing project, repair happens to your organs and tissues during rest. This restorative time is critical to keep your body functioning well and your resistance to illness high. Your body knows what it's doing! The question is this: Will I listen to my body's cues and sleep when I am tired?

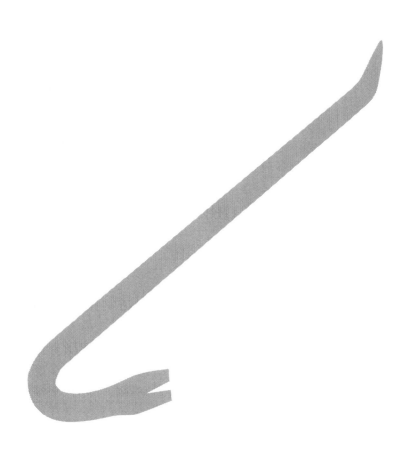

Sleep In The Dark

A nd I mean dark. No nightlight. No blue light coming from the television or clock. No light coming from under the door or through the window. The reason is this: light stimulus disrupts the pineal gland, slowing down the production of melatonin. Melatonin not only helps you sleep, but it regulates hormones, increases immune function and prevents cancer. If making your room completely dark is not possible or practical, wear an eye mask to block the light. You'll not only gain health, you'll feel more rested in the morning. The question is this: What needs to happen for me to sleep in pitch darkness?

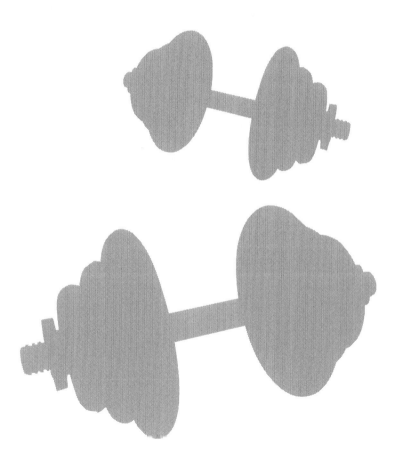

Become A "Morning Person."

The "golden minutes" before midnight (10:00pm–midnight) have the highest quality sleep potential. The habit of going to bed early and waking up early will produce the most long-term health benefits. You can potentially even sleep fewer hours overall, yet feel more rested by going to bed earlier. The bad habit of staying up until after midnight (even if you sleep in late) will eventually affect your vitality. Make yourself a "morning person" and enjoy the benefits of more productivity, better health and fewer bags under your eyes! The question is this: What can I accomplish with an extra hour in the morning?

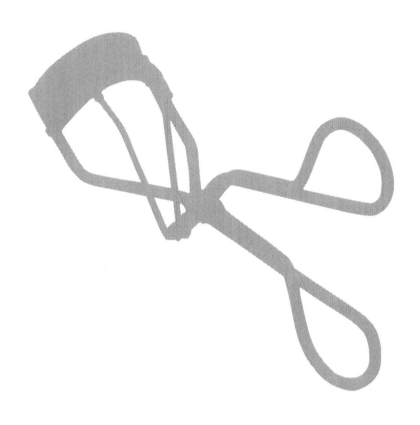

Use The Right Pillow

Finding the right pillow for sleep can prove a challenge, but is worth the effort. To make this task more complicated, proper pillow support needs can change depending on sleeping position. As a general rule, you need more support when sleeping on your side, and none or little while on your back. Consider the space from the tip of your shoulder to your ear. This space needs to be properly filled when sleeping on your side. If your pillow is too thin, you will tend to roll your shoulder forward and tilt your head toward the bed, straining your neck during the night. If you find the tendency to put your hand or arm under your head, that is a sign that your pillow is too thin. If you sleep only on your side, choose an overstuffed or "side sleeper" pillow. For back sleeping, a thin pillow or no pillow is most appropriate to keep the alignment of the ear and shoulder. If you sleep on your side and back, there are pillows that are thicker on the sides with an indent in the center to accommodate both positions. Two more points: avoid stomach sleeping and change your pillow every year. (It will likely flatten over time.) The question is this: Is it time to buy a new pillow?

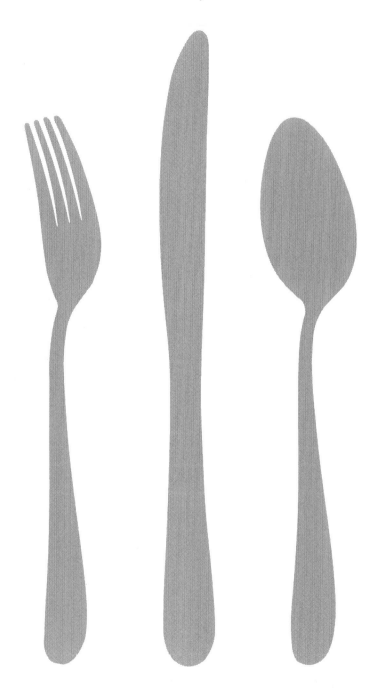

Reduce EMFs In The Bedroom

Power lines, home wiring, computers, appliances, electric blankets, waterbeds and fluorescent lights emit electromagnetic fields (EMFs). Controversial research suggests EMFs may act as a causative factor in brain tumors, leukemia, birth defects, miscarriages, headaches, chronic fatigue, heart problems, stress, forgetfulness and cancer. As a cautious strategy in the bedroom, keep all electrical devices (such as alarm clocks and telephones) at least six feet from your bed. Avoid sleeping under an electric blanket or on a waterbed. Minimally, unplug them before sleeping. (Don't just turn them off.) Ideally, have no wires plugged in near your head (such as behind the headboard). EMFs can disrupt the pineal gland and the production of melatonin and serotonin, which means you don't sleep well or don't wake up rested. You may have noticed sleeping better while camping or during a power outage, which explains we are designed to sleep without any EMFs circling around our bodies. The question is this: What can I unplug?

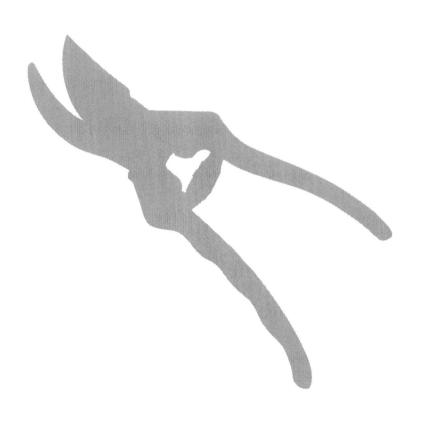

Be "Screen-Free" Before Bed

As we settle into quiet in the evening, the remote or mouse beckons with a magnetic pull. Our mobile phone stays in our hand as we climb under the covers. We become passive as we watch the drama on TV or surf Facebook. Shutting off our brain is a strategy to transition to slumber. Here's another strategy: finish the screen time at least thirty minutes before bed. In that thirty minutes read something. Keep magazines, books and journals on your nightstand. Even just one short chapter in a book will help your brain transition to a healthier sleep. Television, computer and hand-held device screens decrease your production of melatonin, which is the hormone that helps you sleep. Sleep quality improves by finishing screens earlier in the evening. The question is this: What am I reading tonight?

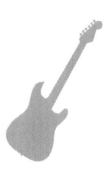

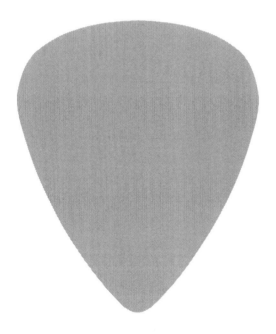

Make Eating Healthy Simple

Want to know the easiest way to determine if a food is healthy for you? You can bet it's healthy if it doesn't come with a food label. Think about it. Whole foods are foods that haven't been processed ... and are close to how they grew naturally. For example, a carrot is a whole food. Your body knows what to do with it. Containing natural digestive enzymes, the carrot is broken down, easily digested, and not stored as fat. Nutritious food generates more life in the body. If the majority of what you eat is whole foods, I guarantee you feel amazingly vital! One idea is to focus on eating primarily salads with a protein source on top. Make a large bowl of salad twice a week. If you keep the lettuce dry, the salad will keep in the refrigerator for at least five days. For each daily salad serving add a protein source (salmon, turkey, beef, hard-boiled egg, walnuts, etc.), and salad dressing. It's simple, healthy, and easy! The question is this: Am I willing to mostly buy foods without labels?

Eat Less

I t may not be the sexiest advice. In fact it's quite boring. To be healthier, more vital and an ideal weight, we need to just eat less. Portion sizes have gotten out of control and, unfortunately, we're getting used to super-sizing. That humongous plate of pasta at our favorite restaurant corresponds to about three meals. Even plate sizes have increased. Here are some great tips for keeping portion size under control: one serving of meat should measure about the size of a deck of cards. A grain serving size equals a tennis ball (1 cup.) Use small plates, bowls, and glassware. Keep your food on the kitchen counter instead of serving it at the table. When grabbing a snack, place the amount you want on a plate instead of holding the whole bag. You might be surprised that you feel just as satisfied with less food, and more energetic! The question is this: Am I willing to eat less to function better?

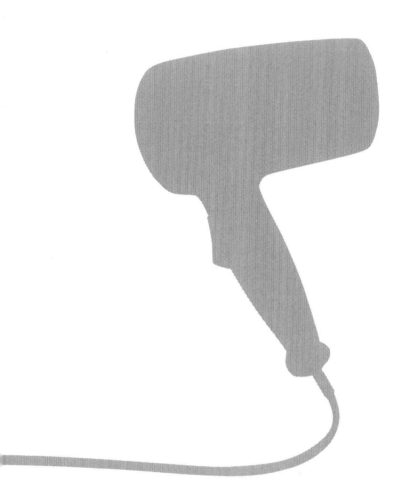

Avoid The Two
Big Bad Ingredients

When my son was three years old, he went on his first play date without me. When I went to pick him up, his playmate's mom told me about a funny interaction she had with Max. She had given him a bagged organic snack. (I think they were cheese crackers.) Max politely handed it back and said, "I can't read yet. Would you please read me the ingredient label?" Amused by his request, she did just that. He thought for a moment and took back the bag saying, "Thank you." Perplexed, the mom asked Max what she could have read that would have made him decide to not eat the snack. He replied, "Well, for starters, high fructose corn syrup or partially hydrogenated vegetable oil." I have educated my son and daughter on why we make the food choices we do, even though I never told him to question his friend's mother! Those two ingredients are, in my opinion, the worst offenders for health. They have been linked with heart disease, osteoporosis, adult-onset diabetes mellitus, weight gain and accelerated aging. The question is this: Am I still buying foods with high fructose corn syrup and partially hydrogenated vegetable oil?

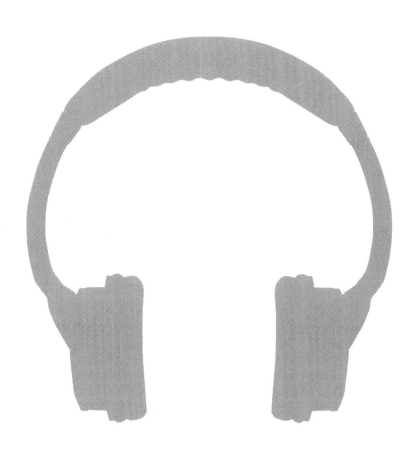

Choose Organic

I had a pre-teen practice member who didn't understand what organic meant. He said it sounded "crunchy and gross!" I kindly asked him what his favorite meal was. He responded that he loved spaghetti and meatballs. I said, "Imagine that your dad just made you that delicious meal from scratch with the finest ingredients he could find. He arranges it beautifully on a plate and sets it in front of you. Right before you eat it though, he mists it with insect killer." Yuck, right? The pre-teen learned that the meal was organic, until his father added the chemicals. He finally got it, and started asking his parents to buy only organic food. But what about price, you ask? Well, here's the most important foods to buy organic (to avoid the biggest load of gross chemicals, preservatives and hormones): meat, milk, coffee, celery, peaches, strawberries, apples, blueberries, nectarines, bell peppers, spinach, kale, cherries, potatoes, and grapes. The question is this: Am I willing to seek out organic to avoid putting chemicals in my body?

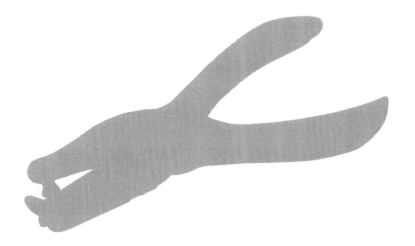

Save The Junk
For Special Occasions

I like a scoop of ice cream as much as the next person, but I don't keep it in the house. Seriously, if "dreamy creamy cookie dough" were in the freezer, I'd eat it. I don't want to ingest dairy and sugar on a daily basis, so I just don't buy it. Doesn't mean I never, ever eat it. Keep the "special" foods special. Buy for only holidays or when in a restaurant. The list, for you, may include ice cream, desserts, special drinks, fried foods, chocolate, and coffee. What you buy, you'll eat. What you see on the pantry shelf, you'll grab. The question is this: Am I eating the junk because I keep buying it?

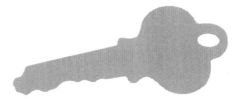

Check For
A Nightshade Sensitivity

D o you love tomatoes, potatoes, eggplant, or colored peppers? They are all part of a class called nightshades and, for some people, can lead to arthritic symptoms and skin problems like eczema. Nightshades contain alkaloids that can impact nerve-muscle function, digestion and joint function in people who are sensitive. That means that if you eat a lot of tomatoes, you may wake up the next morning with stiff and achy joints. Or your child may develop eczema from eating lots of potatoes. Tobacco, belladonna and some over-the-counter pain relievers also contain nightshades. Here's how you figure out if you are sensitive: do a two-week elimination diet. That means for two weeks, eat NO forms of these foods (including ketchup and potato chips, too)! Then for one day, eat a considerable amount of nightshades. Within twenty-four hours you'll know if you have a sensitivity. When I tested this (absolutely not expecting to be sensitive), I woke up the next morning with every single joint in my body hurting, even my fingers. It went away in a few hours, but now I know to not scarf down eggplant parmigiana. Thankfully, a few tomatoes in my salad seem to cause no problem. The question is this: Might I have a nightshade sensitivity?

52 Vitality Tools

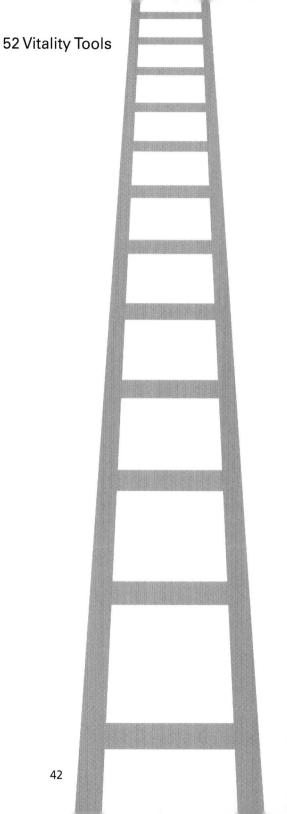

Get Savvy About MSG

If you're thinking, "Oh, right, MSG. It's in cheap Chinese food," then you're not quite savvy yet. MSG, or monosodium glutamate, which contains factory-created free glutamate can also appear under the names yeast extract, calcium or sodium caseinate, autolyzed yeast, protein isolate, autolyzed or hydrolyzed plant or vegetable protein and even natural flavors. Check your favorite food bar, protein powder, or packaged food and see if any of these names come up. MSG is an excitotoxin, which basically means it excites your brain cells to death. Eating too much (or for some people any) MSG will lead to headaches, allergies, and brain tumors. This flavor enhancer is common in fast food. The question is this: Do I know if I am consuming MSG?

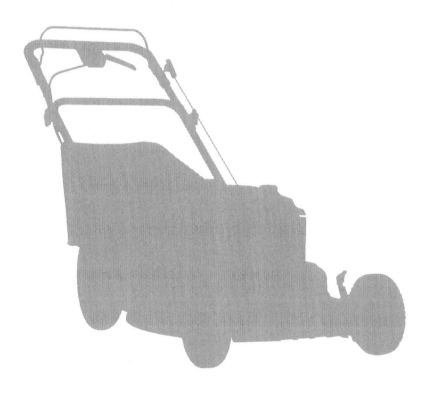

Consider Nutritional Cleansing

"You mean I have to give up wheat, dairy, sugar, caffeine, nightshades, soy, and corn? No way is that possible!" Not only am I telling you it is extremely possible, but the hundreds of people I have led through a one-to-four-week nutritional cleanse have consistently reported results of increased energy, weight loss, improved digestion, resolution of skin problems, and cleared-up sinus congestion. Cleansing works! It works because we are inundated with toxins on a daily basis; toxins that our body struggles to manage. These toxins can be stored in the body, surrounded in mucus. Literally. This mucus is stored in and around our organs, creating puffiness and decreased vitality. A nutritional cleanse gives your body a break, allowing it the opportunity to heal. By eating mainly vegetables, fruits, oats, and brown rice, with some nuts, lentils, all natural meats and healthy fish, the body thrives again. The most common question, by far, at the end of the cleanse is: "Do I have to stop?" Your question, now, is this: Am I willing to eat clean for a few weeks to let my body heal?

Reconsider
The Necessity Of Milk

I am surprised how people still see milk as necessary for bone health. According to Michael Klaper, MD, author of Vegan Nutrition: Pure & Simple, "The human body has no more need for cow's milk than it does for dog's milk, horse's milk, or giraffe's milk." The Dairy Industry has lobbied for the perpetuation of the milk/calcium/bone health myth for decades now. It's becoming evident that the process of homogenization (what turns whole milk into 2% or skim milk) is linked to increased cholesterol and other health problems and pasteurization decreases the absorbability of the calcium in milk. Interestingly, the countries with the highest rates of osteoporosis have the highest consumption of milk. Try broccoli, spinach, oranges, beans and fish, for high-quality, absorbable calcium. Stop leaching the calcium from your bones by avoiding dark carbonated beverages, excess sugar and red meat. The question is this: If I don't need rhinoceros's milk for health, why cow's milk?

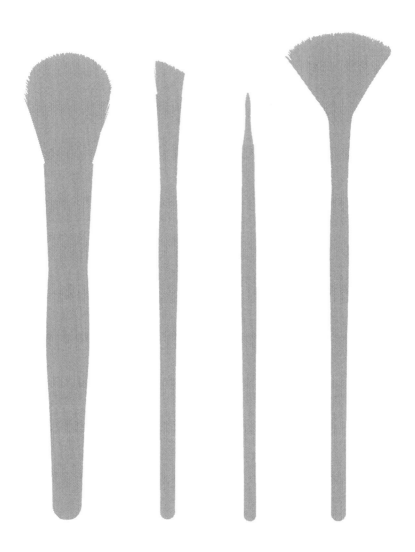

Get A Daily Dose Of Omega-3s

One word that I could use to describe the average American is INFLAMED. Poor food choices, stress, lack of exercise, and our environment create inflammation in the body. This manifests as pain and illness in many different forms. (These maladies include hay fever, depression, diabetes and heart disease.) One reason for this inflammation is a chronic deficiency of omega-3 fatty acids. This has partly happened because our diets consist heavily of omega-6 fatty acids (plant, corn and soy oils). This disrupts the body's inherent necessary balance of omega-3 and omega-6. To create balance, we need to consume more fish, avocados, walnuts, and flax seeds. In addition, I recommend a daily supplement of top-grade fish oil. I've noticed from our practice members that this helps with overall inflammation, pain, achiness, depression, digestion and skin health. The question is this: Am I inflamed?

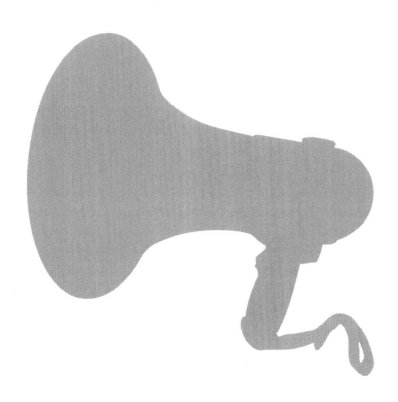

Skip The Sugar

Sugar has no nutritional value. Shocked, aren't you? Seriously though, sugar is in practically everything and comes in many disguises. Sugar hides under the names sucrose, fructose, crystalline fructose, cane sugar, dextrose, corn syrup, high fructose corn syrup (HFCS), sorbitol, malt syrup, maltodextrin, polydextrose and more. We often over-consume this quick-energy substance, leaving the body no choice but to store the excess as fat. That's right. Sugar makes you fat. It also depresses the immune system, so eating any form of sugar while your body works on a "healing project" will set you back. Think of sugar as the "food" for bacteria and viruses. To starve the invader and help your body heal, avoid sugar. The question is this: Does sugar really serve my body in any way?

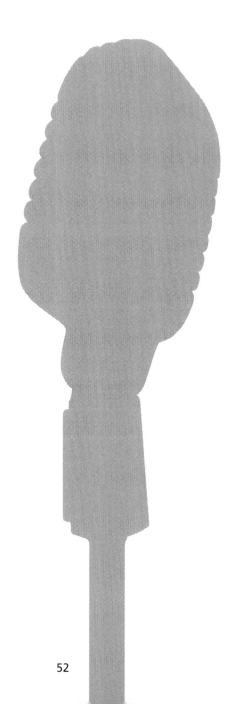

Enjoy Dark Leafy Greens

Kale, spinach, Swiss chard — when I was younger these dark-green leafy plants intimidated and turned me off. I couldn't imagine actually enjoying their consumption. As I've learned more about nutrition and stretched my beliefs, I find that the darker the green, the more nutrient dense, and the more satisfying to eat. The biggest bang for the nutrient buck is these super-star plants. If I had one choice for a class of food to survive on, it would be dark leafy greens. Iron, potassium, calcium, magnesium and most of the great vitamins are packed right in there. Here's my favorite way to prepare them: spinach in salad, kale as kale chips (drizzle with olive oil, sprinkle sea salt and cook flat on a cookie sheet for fifteen minutes at 350 degrees), and Swiss chard sautéed with olive oil, garlic and onions. Just thinking about it right now makes me hungry for the nutrient boost. The question is this: Have I tried dark leafy greens lately?

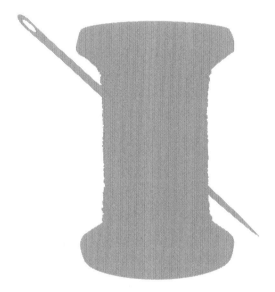

Sip Water All Day

Do you notice dry mouth and thirst first thing in the morning? Chronic dehydration zaps your energy, health and vitality. Alcohol, high protein intake, eating mostly processed food, sweating, and not enough water are common everyday causes of dehydration. Here's the best way to start counteracting dehydration: sip water all day long. Your body can only absorb about four ounces of water every thirty minutes, so sipping about a "Dixie cup" every half hour will keep you the most hydrated. I recommend finding a special water container to have next to you at all times. If water doesn't appeal to you, try adding fresh lemon or lime. The alkalizing effect of lemon is healthy and the sweet taste encourages you to drink more often. Here's a buying tip: the thinner the lemon skin, the sweeter the lemon (with a higher mineral content). The main benefits you'll notice from proper hydration include fat loss, revitalized energy, a younger appearance, reduced blood pressure, less joint pain and improved bowel movements. The question is this: Am I hydrated?

Dr. Jenny Bruck

Feed Your Brain
With Movement

Move it, don't lose it! The brain and movement are more intimately connected than most people realize. What I mean is that when you move (walk, hop, skip or run), you literally provide "nutrients" to the brain. The vermis of the cerebellum is the part of the brain that processes movement and processes learning, decision making, and attention. This means that when you sit all day (drive to work, sit at a computer, drive home, then sit on the couch and watch TV), you don't feed your brain! As humans, we are meant to move… and we often forget that in today's world. I challenge you to move! The question is this: Am I stimulating my brain with movement?

Move Your Joints

You begin to degenerate any joint that you don't move on a daily basis. This means that moving your joints (spine, hips, knees, ankles, shoulders, elbows and wrists, for example) helps avoid arthritic symptoms. With today's lifestyle, if you mainly sit and walk, as compared to doing more complex movements you might see in yoga for example, you will build an arthritic body over time. Moving the joints in as many ways as possible on a daily basis will keep them lubricated and healthy. I recommend regular stretching, yoga, dance, martial arts, or any other form of dynamic full-body exercise. In addition, the spine needs to be able to properly move each joint from your neck to your tailbone. If one of these joints gets "locked" or subluxated, a chiropractor helps to restore proper motion to the spine. Because you don't necessarily feel subluxation, regular visits to a chiropractor are a smart choice for healthcare. The question is this: Am I moving all my joints?

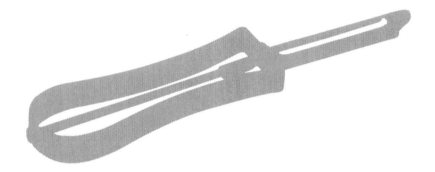

See Exercise As An Essential Nutrient

Often, we hear people say they will exercise when they "get around to it," or "have more time." Our culture sees exercise as a chore to be done in a specific location. Additionally, we tend to view exercise as optional for health and a luxury for people with time or ability. Movement, in the form of exercise, is so much more valuable than for just weight loss, improved athletic performance, or improving the way we look. Exercise is a requirement for normal physiology and health. Redefine what exercise means to you and consider how to enjoy more movement. This may mean taking the stairs instead of the elevator, riding your bike instead of driving, and going for a walk on your lunch break. In fact, you might be surprised how much more energetic, dynamic and vital you feel with increased movement. The question is this: How can I move more?

Make Exercise Who You Are

If your current belief system is that exercise requires willpower, amazing discipline, or giving up something (your time, energy, comfort), then you will likely fail at making it a regular part of your life. One way to think differently is this: make exercise not something you try to do, but who you are. Many years ago, I decided to start jogging. I never saw myself as a runner, and didn't necessarily have a natural aptitude for the activity. In fact, I struggled to enjoy it. Wanting to press forward, I decided that I wasn't trying to run, but I was a runner. I would actually say this to others. "Oh, on Tuesday morning I'll be exercising. I'm a runner." This subtle change in my perception helped me to continue to incorporate jogging into my life. Eventually, with consistent effort, I began to enjoy the sport. The same can go for any form of exercise. The question is this: Am I someone who exercises?

52 Vitality Tools

Work Smart At The Computer

Most people these days can't escape it: workstation subluxation. This refers to the body misalignments that happen from sitting at a computer. You know what I mean — your elbow or wrist starts to throb, your shoulders ache, your neck feels tight, your energy depletes, and your eyes feel strained. We are absolutely not designed to endure this type of stress, particularly for hours a day. There is something you can do to ease the burden. In fact, I consider this a must if you want to experience vitality. Set up your computer as ergonomically as possible. Have the middle of the screen level with your eyes. Relax your shoulders and bend your arms ninety degrees while keeping your elbows at your sides; this is where the keyboard and mouse should be. Your chair should be comfortable, allowing a natural curve to the lower back and feet firmly on the floor. When working on a laptop computer, use a separate keyboard and mouse to avoid strain. Additionally, you may need to raise the laptop on a stand to elevate the screen. The time, money and effort it takes to accomplish this task is more than worth it. The question is this: Is my computer set up correctly for my body?

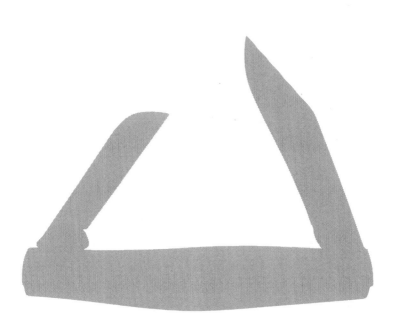

Dr. Jenny Bruck

Take Frequent
"Screen" Breaks

Media screens are an abundant part of our culture. We have screens in cars, on our phones and a television or computer in every room of our home. We rely on media for news, communication, school, and work. We may have an awareness of the potential health consequences of prolonged screen use for children, but rarely do we see adults consciously monitor their own bodies in relation to screen use. We are less aware of the emotional, mental, and physical consequences of being plugged in for hours a day. Just take an unplugged vacation (it was necessary for me to go to a Mexican "eco resort" without electricity to accomplish this), and you can experience how we are truly meant to feel. Seriously, people are numb to what living should actually feel like. A hike in nature is another way to experience the phenomenon of being unplugged. Here's a lesser, maybe more doable, option for your daily life: take a ten-minute break every hour. Go for a walk around the office, get some fresh air, look at something far away (to reduce eye strain), stretch your body and take some deep breaths. The question is this: When was the last time I really unplugged?

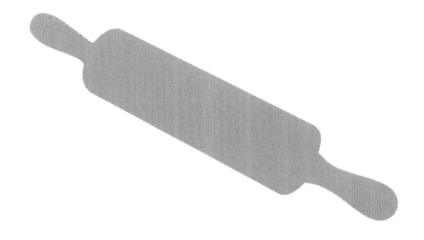

Keep Your Head Up

An epidemic is affecting the vitalism of our community. It is often associated with elderly, frail people, but can be seen as early as age six. It is called Forward Head Syndrome (FHS). The proper alignment is easy to picture: looking at a person from the side, the earlobe should line up above the tip of the shoulder. When the head goes forward, the person appears unhealthy and older, often with a hump in the upper back. Other than discomfort and pain, this "hunchback" appearance (which can significantly increase the likelihood of death according to the American Geriatrics Society) has dire health consequences. FHS adds up to 30 pounds of abnormal weight to the neck bones. It can deplete lung capacity by up to 30%, leading to heart and blood problems. The large intestine loses good bowel function. There is even a correlation with uterine prolapse. To detect and work on FHS, see a chiropractor, for this is likely a structural problem, not laziness. The question is this: Are my ears in front of my shoulder?

(Rejuvenation Strategy, Dr. Rene Cailliet, director of the Dept. of Physical Medicine and Rehabilitation at the U. of So. California)

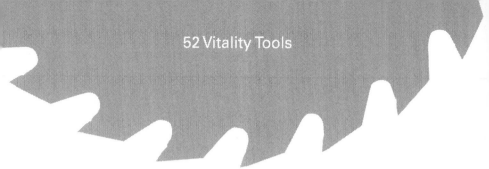

Put On Some Muscle

The average person gains twenty pounds between the ages of 25 and 55. We also tend to lose muscle mass as we age. So basically, we lose muscle and replace it with fat! This is not your destiny if you are determined to put on some muscle. Just eating less without weight-bearing exercise will cause you to lose fat and muscle. When the weight is gained back (which it often is), you gain back fat. This creates a slower metabolism and a person who says, "I barely eat and I still can't get to a healthy weight." This happens because fat burns seventy times fewer calories than muscle. The way to look better, feel better, live longer, and keep a healthy weight? Gain muscle! Assuming you're eating a healthy diet, gaining muscle will keep you vital. How? Choose a variety of weight-bearing movement like weight lifting, yoga, sports, dancing, etc. The question is this: Have I done a push-up lately?

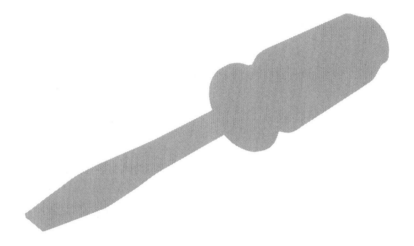

Breathe Right

I was in yoga class and my instructor, Erin, taught me how to breathe. I know what you're thinking, "Um, I know how to breathe!" Listen to me: you may not be doing it right! I certainly wasn't. Put your hand on your belly. Now, breathe in. If the air reaches only to your lower neck or collarbones, you're breathing too shallowly. This is common, especially with people who sit a lot. Breathe deeper and work to inhale the air to fill your lungs, even the bottom corners. Now try again and see if you can fill your "belly." With your hand still there, notice your belly expand as you breathe in. Here's where it gets really interesting. Some of you, like me, may experience that when you breathe deep into your belly that your belly doesn't go out, but in. That is reverse breathing. Work to correct it, allowing your belly to go in as you exhale. Practicing this exercise daily will oxygenate your brain, give you energy, and keep you vital! The question is this: Am I breathing right?

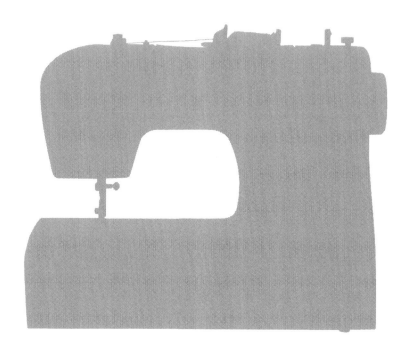

Exercise Smart

The amount of oxygen you're able to breathe per minute is directly tied to your metabolism, specifically the number of calories you burn per minute. More oxygen = more efficient metabolism. There are smart ways to exercise that will significantly increase your oxygen intake. Specifically, interval training will increase muscle mass and oxygen intake. Interval training means you have short bursts of high-intensity exercise, followed by longer periods of lighter exercise. For example, while out for a walk or jog, you could periodically sprint. These bursts help you get so much more out of your workout! The question is this: How can I exercise smarter?

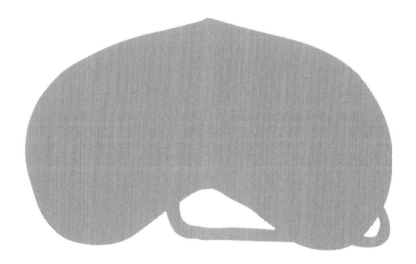

Reduce Repetitive Strain

You may know the best body positions for sleep, computer use and work but forget them when you get extremely focused on a task or feel stressed. I fully relate to this. For example, when I get extra busy and am focusing intently on patients, I tend to forget about my body positioning while adjusting. An hour can go by before I realize I have been slightly straining myself. If I keep this up too long, I ache by the end of the week. Maybe this has happened to your elbow or wrist from prolonged computer work, to your lower back after eighteen great holes of golf, or to your shoulders after two hours into a riveting video game. It's one thing to feel the strain and to stop and rest. It's another to be mindful enough to prevent the strain. Periodically "checking-in" with your body position and movement is a simple task that will contribute considerably to vitality. Here's a more specific suggestion: when doing a repetitive task (computer use, driving, cleaning, a sport or hobby, etc.) stop half-way through and change positions. Move your body around and get a sense of how comfortable you feel. If you feel stiff, lethargic or in pain, take a moment to drink water, stretch and rest. The question is this: When can I reduce body strain?

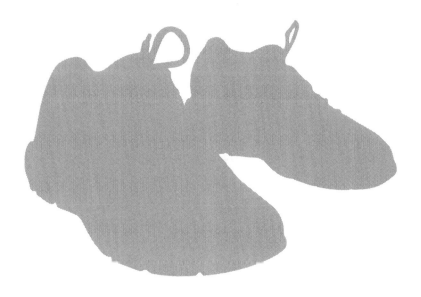

Let Go Of The Stress

Stress changes your body chemistry. It puts you into fight-or-flight mode — even just perceiving stress with your thoughts. For example, if as you trekked through the jungle, a tiger charged at you, you would secrete adrenalin and cortisol to help you run away fast. Now, even lying quietly in bed at night and thinking about the tiger charging you (or the bills that need to be paid, or a hurtful relationship, or a the story you keep replaying from your past) will create the same body chemistry. If you sink into this state often enough, it will wreak havoc on your body! How to counteract this chemical stew? Say what you need to say. Do what you need to do. Fix what you perceive causes you to feel stress. In the meantime, take a moment during the day to sit quietly and clear your mind–just allow yourself to feel love. Change your body chemistry. The question is this: Can I remember that, ultimately, there is no tiger?

Forgive

Holding back forgiveness, for others or yourself, creates a burden on your shoulders. This burden mostly hurts you. Imagine letting go of that emotional weight. One simple way to do this is to write a letter. Pour out your heart and forgive. You don't have to do anything with the letter. You could even burn it. Not only will you feel better, but on a physical level, you may notice recurring symptoms go away. Pain and discomforts may lessen. You will physically look lighter, softer, less worried, and less anxious. You may even regain a "spark" that you once had. This shows in your face, skin, and body language. People will be more attracted to your renewed energy, making communication easier. You have nothing to lose by forgiving. The question is this: Who can I forgive?

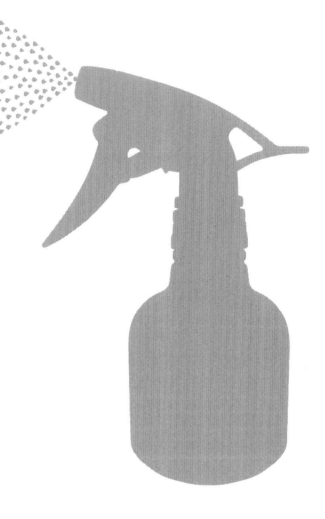

Do What You Love

Take the time to consider what inspires you. Maybe it's painting, playing baseball, dancing, lunch with friends, swimming in the ocean, or organizing closets. (Yes, some people enjoy organizing closets.) What do you really, really love to do? To discover this, you may need to think back over your life and ponder the moments when you felt most alive, energized and happy. Once you find that special something, schedule it. I mean it. Write down in your calendar: "Wednesday 12:30–1:00 pm swing in hammock." As silly as that may seem, the anticipation and joy it brings to your life will carry you through the mundane tasks. The question is this: What do I love to do?

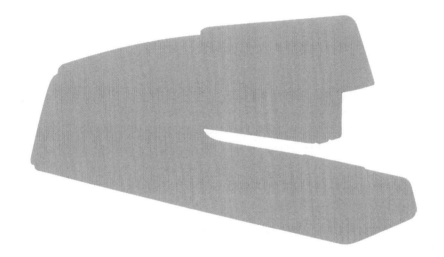

Give A New Habit
Time To Stick

Your body responds well to rhythm. Like a toddler, you function best when you go to bed and wake up at the same time each day. Eating breakfast each morning, flossing your teeth every day, stretching your muscles each evening: all healthy habits. It's common to flow in and out of healthy habits over a lifetime. What matters most is that you can get back to your vitality-creating choices when you fall off. On average, it takes twenty-one days to fully develop a new habit. So stick to going to the gym, eating a salad daily, or drinking lots of water — eventually it will feel easy. Once it's a habit, it becomes who you are. The question is this: What is worth twenty-one days of my time to become a new habit?

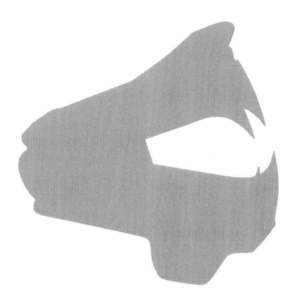

Borrow My Mantra

Have you ever read a line in a book and it hits you right in the heart? You re-read it over and over and feel a connection, as if you had written the line yourself. This happened to me when I read the book Creative Visualization by Shakti Gawain. She wrote the visualization, "Everything is coming to me easily and effortlessly." This mind strategy has served me well. I have successfully used this mantra when rock climbing, taming a toddler's tantrum, and public speaking. When something feels hard, I remember that (oh, yeah!) everything comes to me easily and effortlessly. I have the phrase "easy and effortless" mentally tattooed in my mind. The result? A ridiculous number of people ask me why things seem so easy for me, why I am so lucky, and what my secret is. There. I've told you my secret. Feel free to use it. The question is this: Why not just remind myself that everything is easy and effortless?

Schedule Time To Work On You

We live in a fast-paced world. Time can go by in the blink of an eye, and that time may be mostly filled with laundry, dishes, errands, deadlines and sleep. The most vital people I know take the time for self-care. For some, self-care is as simple as a timely haircut, clipping their nails, and rubbing lotion on their face. For others, a hair "blow-out," manicure and facial are the standard they want to achieve. Whatever your level of grooming, make sure you take the time to schedule it and pamper yourself. It's amazing what a difference a small amount of additional self-care can do to improve self-esteem! You are worth it...and you deserve to make time for you as important as your dog's monthly pet grooming (I laugh as I write this, because I know that this happens!) The question is this: What can I schedule for me to feel great?

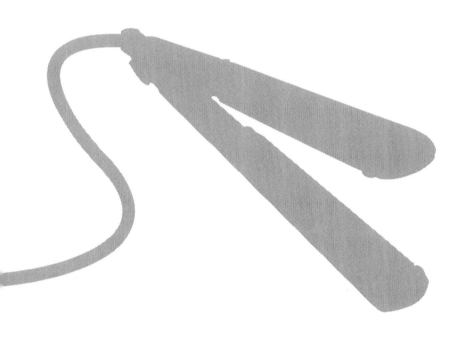

Choose Words That Serve You

I can, I choose, I wish, I will, I am, thank you! We are more responsive to others when they respond with "yes" words or words of positive affirmation. As soon as someone says "I can't" or "I won't," we feel a subconscious contraction of spirit. The world responds to us in the same way. When we use expansive, life-affirming words, we draw more energy and abundance to our life. And perhaps, most importantly, it just feels better. Here's an example: instead of saying, "I can't afford that!" say, "I am choosing to spend my money in different ways." Sure, maybe it's on the rent or your car payment, but it is a choice that you make, and a wise choice. Here's another example. Imagine scheduling a lunch date with a friend. Instead of, "I can't do any time this week," how about, "I can do next week better if that works for you." The question is this: Can I better monitor my words to feel good?

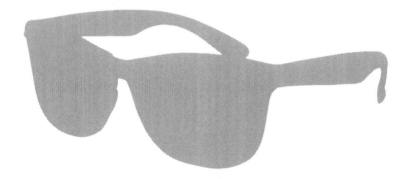

Let Go Of Limitations

Mary Kay Ash said, "Aerodynamically the bumblebee shouldn't be able to fly, but the bumblebee doesn't know that so it goes on flying anyway." We see this all the time in children. They charge ahead with no fear because they don't have a preconceived idea about their abilities (until we, as parents, place it on them). I wonder how much more we could create, accomplish and manifest if we didn't see any limitations. We hear fabulous stories about people who overcame tremendous odds to go from poor to rich, wheelchair-bound to running, and grossly obese to fit. What they likely had in common was not only drive, but also the decision see no limits. The question is this: What would I attempt to do if I knew I could not fail? (1)

1. Robert H. Schuller can be credited with originating this question in his 1973 book *"You Can Become the Person You Want To Be."*

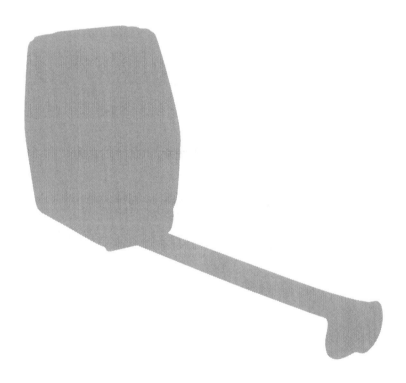

Open Your Heart

J ack Kornfield said, "We don't have to improve ourselves, we just have to let go of what blocks our heart." I think of a challenge our young daughter had in kindergarten with the class "bully." Shortly after she had seen the movie The Grinch Who Stole Christmas, her teacher told us how Mackenzie had befriended the struggling child and was helping him integrate better with the class. I asked Mackenzie what had happened and she said, "I decided to help make his heart bigger." Loving ourselves and others, unconditionally, allows pain, sorrow, anger and fear to melt away. An institute called HeartMath (www.heartmath.org) has studied how electromagnetic forces of our heart radiate as much as 15 feet around us. When our energies are low and negative, we affect others in our proximity in a negative way. Conversely, we help make someone's heart "bigger" when we come from feelings of love. The question is this: How big is my heart?

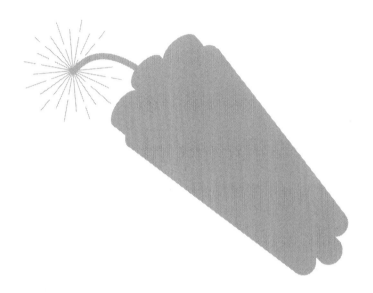

Remember Your Future Is Undecided

L ife can turn on a dime. Security is an illusion and personal growth is never fully realized. That is the curse and the beauty of life. We never "finally make it" while we're still alive, because there is always the next step, the next day. I recently read in Earl Nightingale's book *Lead the Field* about how the path of achieving a goal is the success, not the achievement of the goal. I had heard this quote when I was younger, but it finally sank in as I was able to look back on my life and see how achieving a goal was not what brought me happiness. Happiness is being in the moment, every moment, while working towards what you want. Despite your past circumstances, each day presents an opportunity for you to express love, accomplish your goals and experience life. Abraham Lincoln said, "The best way to predict your future is to create it." The question is this: What are you creating of yourself today?

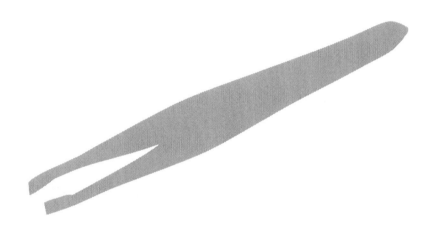

Live From Your Values

One of the most life-changing seminars I've ever attended was with Dr. John DeMartini. There was an exercise to determine values (available at www.drdemartini.com). He asked questions like, "What do I think about and talk about the most?" and "Where do I spend my time, energy and money?" The intention is to pinpoint what is truly most important. Our true values may be different than societal expectations. An (albeit stereotypical) example is: some women are living their dream by staying home to raise children. Others find that without an outlet of work or a hobby, they are not fulfilled, despite how much they love their family. Aligning our life with our values will help us to feel the most vital. When we live a life that is incongruent to our highest values, we are likely living the life that someone else wants us to live or that we grew up thinking we should live. The question is this: What are my values?

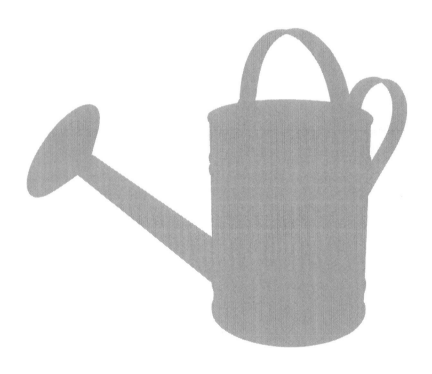

Clear The Clutter

Clutter is not separate from you. However, you are also not your clutter. This applies to mind clutter as well as physical clutter. Neither serves you. The clutter in your garage had to begin somewhere, possibly in your mind? Examine what thought processes lead to clutter: holding on to what you don't need, procrastination that you'll deal with it later, rebelling against being told what to do, or feeling it's not worth doing if it can't be done perfectly. Whether it's drawers full of junk or a head full of fear, clutter disables our ability to move forward. Start with what feels easy: maybe a space on your desk, your pocketbook or the passenger's seat of your car. Start somewhere. As your physical space clears, watch how you feel. Better, isn't it? The question is this: Where is my broom?

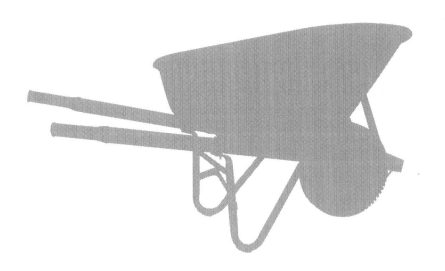

Focus On What You Want

I treasure the expression energy flows where focus goes. How true this is! The assertion especially relates to health and vitality. I had a practice member decide to start eating better. After attending my nutrition workshop, he began investing more energy in how he fueled his body. He took more time in the grocery store, read labels, and ruminated on what meals to prepare. The result: after just a few weeks he had dropped eight pounds and was completely re-energized! Here's another example: I wanted more public speaking opportunities, so I focused on it. Not only did I think and talk more about speaking; I made a vision board, journaled, and invested in speaking products and tools. Within a month, I had acquired four new speaking opportunities and an interview for a major speaking gig. My focus on what I wanted created more energy, and more results. You want to change your image? Focus on it. You want to become a better listener? Focus on it. You want to make more money? Focus, focus, focus. This may mean taking action, talking more about it or learning more. As long as you persist and create positive feelings about what you are focusing on, I believe you attract it. The question is this: Where is my focus?

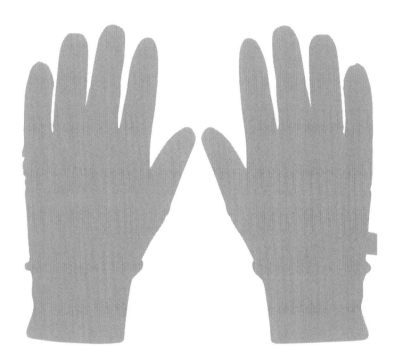

Slow Down To Think

Are you quick to take action? Some people, like me, live by the quote: "the difference between someone who is successful and someone who is not, is people who are successful do. That's it." Being a "doer" often serves people well. It's often a habit to muscle through and create what you want. This act of control and power, however, is often inefficient and energy draining. Purposefully slowing down to ponder before taking action is brilliance. Literally sit down, stop working, and just think. Think as big as you can. Imagine the most fulfilling reasons, outcomes and possibilities. Develop a system. It's not always easy to slow down. In fact, in some ways it is harder than "doing." The benefit, though, is worth it. This could pertain to how you organize your closet, clean your home, buy holiday gifts, manage money, or create time with family. When we live haphazardly, we create stress. When we live purposefully, we create vitality. The question is this: What can I ponder?

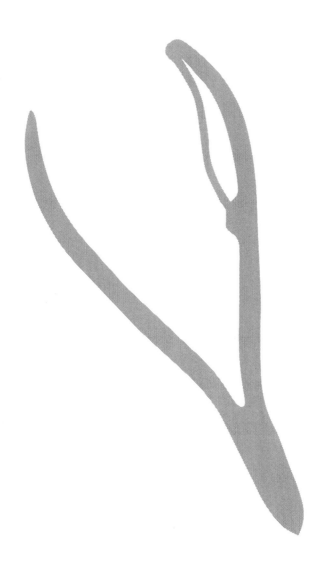

Bonus Tool

Smile

I was at a beauty salon the other day and saw a pretty woman, about forty years old, who was getting the works: hair extensions, a manicure, eyebrow waxing, and a make-up lesson. She appeared to put significant value, effort and money into her appearance. The only thing is, she didn't smile. I noticed her frown lines and the look of strain in her face more than her expensive hair and clothing. Instead of being captivated by her beauty, I was repelled by her countenance. Consider smiling more, even when you don't feel like it. Interestingly, smiling may improve your mood, so the old adage "fake it until you make it" actually applies. Try this: smile when alone. Smile in the shower, while driving and even when falling asleep. By lifting the face, smiling makes you look younger. Smile often, and the "smile lines" you create will make you appear younger even when you're not smiling. Magnetically engaging others with a genuine grin is free, easy and energizing. The question is this: Am I building frown lines or smile lines today?

52 Vitality Tools

Acknowledgements

The space in my life to write this book opened and then closed many times over several years. When it was a priority, I found myself tucked away at Hilltop Café in Wilton, NH, enjoying the quiet hum while focusing on these pages. My children, Max and Kenzie, knew mom was "up at the café" writing. As a working mother, their unconditional love has kept me sane. I hope one day they will enjoy this little book for its content, despite its author.

Thank you to my editor Sylvie Kurtz for the exciting process of critiquing my book. I loved the back and forth exchange, pushing me to become a better writer. Also to John Lewis and Dr. Allen Miner for another layer of editing and valuable insight.

I have had a long professional relationship with the talented Mark Plamondon, a marketing copywriter and graphic designer. For over seventeen years he has kept my practice looking fantastic with custom printed posters and handouts. When I asked him to be the Creative Director for this book, he not only agreed, he brought passion and intensity to the project. He is responsible for the cover design, all illustrations, book layout and the needed push to bring it to completion. Mark, you are forever in my gratitude.

Seriously, Alyssa Havens, can your photography be any more fantastic? Thank you for the cover photo, and for documenting my life with beautiful pictures.

In the final manuscript reviews, it dawned on me that this book was possible because of two extremely influential people in my life. My sister, Dr. Robin Bruck, set me on the path to

Acknowledgements

health and vitality. By example and by her loving nature, she has always pointed me in the best direction for personal growth. Early in my career I was fortunate to meet Dr. C.J. Mertz. His mentoring not only greatly shaped my life and practice, it is the basis for many tools outlined in this book. My heart will always overflow with appreciation for you both.

Finally, there are hundreds of people that drive me to get out of bed every day and perpetuate vitality. My sincere hugs and high-fives to the team and practice members of SCC.

Eat, Move, Rest, Think and Play Your Way to Abundant Vitality

- Wake up every morning relaxed, confident and eager to start the day.

- Feel a constant supply of energy.

- Learn cool stuff like — *get this* — sunshine is actually GOOD for us. *(Details inside.)*

- Delve deeper into vitality topics of particular interest to reap maximum benefits.

- Listen as vitality expert and professional speaker Dr. Jenny Bruck shares secrets that if used wisely could help you attain your dreams.

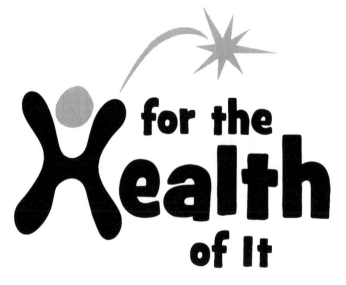

for the

Xealth
of It

Raw Talk About Full Potential Living

Discover a FUN, FREE, and EASY Resource that Promises You a Roadmap to Heightened Health and Vitality

In *52 Vitality Tools* Dr. Jenny encapsulates many facets of vitality. You get the essence and a path is suggested. Often that's all you need.

But if you're inquisitive you'll sometimes want to know more. Fill in the details. Tune in to

- http://ForTheHealthOfIt.podbean.com

In her shows Dr. Jenny explains the how and why of things in simple straightforward ways that occur to only those with real understanding.

If you're working on a strategy to reach *your* full potential Dr. Jenny's podcast can help you get there.

The name of Dr. Jenny's online radio-style show is — as you might have guessed — "For The Health Of It."

- http://ForTheHealthOfIt.podbean.com

The shows are informal, mostly unscripted, and absolutely spot-on. Each podcast runs about 25 min.; feels like less.

Bountiful rewards await. Is now a good time?

Why not check out Dr. Jenny's podcast *now* and bookmark the invaluable FREE resource while you're there?

http://ForTheHealthOfIt.podbean.com

Notes

_____

_____

_____

_____

_____

_____

_____

_____

_____

_____

_____

_____

_____

_____

_____

_____

_____

_____

_____

_____

_____

_____

Notes

Notes

_____

_____

_____

_____

_____

_____

_____

_____

_____

_____

_____

_____

_____

_____

_____

_____

_____

_____

_____

_____

_____

_____

WANT TO LEARN MORE? GO TO
http://ForTheHealthOfIt.podbean.com

Notes

WANT TO LEARN MORE? GO TO
http://ForTheHealthOfIt.podbean.com

Notes

_____

_____

_____

_____

_____

_____

_____

_____

_____

_____

_____

_____

_____

_____

_____

_____

_____

_____

_____

_____

WANT TO LEARN MORE? GO TO
http://ForTheHealthOfIt.podbean.com